Osteoporosis Diet Cookbook for Beginners

A Step-by-Step Guide to Bone-Strengthening Meals

Ennis James

Copyright © 2024 by **Ennis James**
All rights reserved

No part of this publication may be reproduced, stored in a retrieval system, or transmitted, in any form or by any means, electronic, mechanical, photocopying, recording, or otherwise, without the prior written permission of the author.

The information in this ebook is true and complete to the best of our knowledge. All recommendation are made without guarantee on the part of author or publisher. The author and publisher disclaim any liability in connection with the use of this information.

Table of Contents

Introduction — 4
    Understanding Osteoporosis — 8
    What is Osteoporosis? — 11
    Importance of Diet in Managing Osteoporosis — 14

Chapter 1: Breakfast Recipes — 17
    Calcium-Rich Smoothie — 17
    Spinach and Feta Omelet — 19
    Greek Yogurt with Almonds and Berries — 21
    Fortified Oatmeal with Flaxseeds — 23
    Cottage Cheese and Pineapple Bowl — 25
    Whole Grain Toast with Avocado and Sesame Seeds — 27
    Chia Seed Pudding with Blueberries — 29
    Scrambled Eggs with Kale and Mushrooms — 31
    Buckwheat Pancakes with Fresh Fruit — 33
    Quinoa Breakfast Bowl with Nuts and Dried Fruits — 35

Chapter 2: Lunch Recipes — 37
    Grilled Chicken Salad with Spinach and Walnuts — 37
    Quinoa and Black Bean Salad — 39
    Salmon and Avocado Wrap — 41
    Lentil Soup with Kale — 43
    Chickpea and Tomato Salad — 45
    Tofu Stir-Fry with Broccoli and Sesame — 47
    Tuna Salad with Mixed Greens — 49

Sweet Potato and Black Bean Burrito Bowl	51
Turkey and Swiss Lettuce Wraps	53
Mediterranean Farro Salad	55
Chapter 3: Dinner Recipes	**57**
Baked Cod with Asparagus	57
Stuffed Bell Peppers with Quinoa and Turkey	59
Spinach and Ricotta Stuffed Chicken Breast	61
Grilled Salmon with Avocado Salsa	63
Beef and Broccoli Stir-Fry	65
Baked Eggplant Parmesan	67
Lemon Garlic Shrimp with Brown Rice	70
Pork Tenderloin with Apple Slaw	72
Vegetable and Chickpea Curry	74
Mushroom and Barley Risotto	76
Chapter 4: Desserts	**78**
Baked Apples with Cinnamon	78
Chia Seed Pudding with Mango	80
Dark Chocolate Almond Bark	82
Berry Yogurt Popsicles	84
Oatmeal Raisin Cookies	86
Conclusion	**88**

Introduction

Sarah had always been the picture of health. An avid runner and yoga enthusiast, she never imagined her bones might betray her. But at 55, after a minor fall led to a fractured wrist, her doctor delivered an unexpected diagnosis: osteoporosis.

Confused and a bit scared, Sarah turned to the internet for answers. She discovered a wealth of information, but it was overwhelming and often contradictory. She needed a clear, practical guide to help her manage her condition through diet. That's when she stumbled upon the "Osteoporosis Diet Cookbook for Beginners."

Curious, she read the description: "A comprehensive guide to building strong bones and improving overall health through delicious, easy-to-make recipes." It sounded perfect, but Sarah was skeptical. Could a cookbook really make that much of a difference?

Sarah decided to give it a try. When the book arrived, she was immediately impressed by its user-friendly layout. The introduction provided a clear understanding of osteoporosis, its causes, and why diet is crucial in managing the disease. She appreciated the emphasis on practical advice, like setting up a bone-healthy kitchen and essential cooking tools.

The breakfast section caught her eye first. Sarah had always believed breakfast was the most important meal of the day, but she had no idea how much impact it could have on her bone health. The cookbook offered a variety of delicious options, from a Calcium-Rich Smoothie to Buckwheat Pancakes with Fresh Fruit. Each recipe was accompanied by detailed nutritional information, so she knew exactly how it would benefit her bones.

Excited to start her new journey, Sarah tried the Greek Yogurt with Almonds and Berries the next morning. It was simple to prepare, and the taste was delightful. More importantly, she felt empowered knowing she was taking a positive step toward strengthening her bones.

As the weeks went by, Sarah found herself eagerly exploring the lunch and dinner sections. The Grilled Chicken Salad with Spinach and Walnuts became a lunchtime favorite, while the Baked Cod with Asparagus was a hit at dinner. Each recipe was designed with bone health in mind, rich in calcium, vitamin D, and other essential nutrients.

The cookbook also included snacks and smoothies, perfect for those moments when Sarah needed a quick, nutritious bite. She loved the Almond Butter Apple Slices and the refreshing Green Goddess Smoothie. These options kept her energized throughout the day without compromising her bone health.

Sarah was pleasantly surprised by the dessert section. She had a sweet tooth, and the thought of giving up treats was daunting. But the cookbook offered healthy alternatives like Baked Apples with Cinnamon and Dark Chocolate Almond Bark. These desserts were not only delicious but also contributed to her overall health.

Meal planning and preparation tips were another highlight. Sarah appreciated the sample meal plans and shopping list guide, which made grocery trips more efficient. The cookbook even provided cooking techniques to preserve nutrients, ensuring she got the most out of every meal.

Beyond recipes, the "Osteoporosis Diet Cookbook for Beginners" offered lifestyle tips. It emphasized the importance of exercise, sunlight for vitamin D, and avoiding smoking and excessive alcohol. It was a holistic approach that complemented Sarah's dietary changes perfectly.

Three months into using the cookbook, Sarah had a follow-up appointment with her doctor. Her bone density had improved, and she felt stronger and more vibrant. Her doctor was impressed and asked what she had been doing differently. Sarah proudly mentioned the cookbook and how it had revolutionized her diet and lifestyle.

The "Osteoporosis Diet Cookbook for Beginners" was more than just a collection of recipes. It was a lifeline, a guide that empowered Sarah to take control of her health in a way she never thought possible. It was practical, easy to follow, and most importantly, it worked.

For anyone diagnosed with osteoporosis or looking to prevent it, this cookbook was a game-changer. It wasn't just about food; it was about transforming lives, one delicious meal at a time. Sarah couldn't recommend it enough. It had given her hope, strength, and a renewed zest for life. And that, she believed, was worth every penny.

Understanding Osteoporosis

Osteoporosis is a condition characterized by weakened bones, which increases the risk of fractures. It often develops silently over the years, only becoming apparent when a minor fall or even a sudden movement results in a broken bone. The bones most commonly affected are the hip, spine, and wrist, but osteoporosis can affect any bone in the body. This condition is particularly prevalent among older adults, especially postmenopausal women, due to the drop in estrogen levels, which plays a crucial role in maintaining bone density. Men are also at risk, though typically at an older age than women.

The development of osteoporosis is influenced by a combination of genetic, lifestyle, and environmental factors. A family history of the condition can significantly increase your risk, as can certain medical conditions and medications. Lifestyle choices, such as smoking, excessive alcohol consumption, and a sedentary lifestyle, also contribute to the weakening of bones. Moreover, inadequate intake of calcium and vitamin D, essential nutrients for bone health, is a major factor that accelerates bone density loss.

Nutrition plays a pivotal role in both the prevention and management of osteoporosis. A diet rich in calcium and vitamin D is essential for maintaining healthy bones. Calcium is the primary building block of bone tissue, while vitamin D helps the body absorb calcium more efficiently. Foods high in calcium include dairy products like milk, cheese, and yogurt, as well as leafy green vegetables, almonds, and fortified foods. Vitamin D can be obtained from fatty fish, egg yolks, fortified foods, and sunlight exposure.

In addition to calcium and vitamin D, other nutrients are essential for bone health. Magnesium, potassium, and vitamin K are important for bone strength and mineralization. Protein is also crucial as it makes up a significant part of bone tissue. However, it's important to balance protein intake, as excessive protein can increase calcium loss. An osteoporosis diet should include a variety of foods to ensure all these nutrients are adequately supplied.

Managing osteoporosis through diet involves more than just increasing calcium and vitamin D intake. It also requires reducing the consumption of foods and substances that can harm bone health. Excessive salt, caffeine, and alcohol can interfere with the body's ability to absorb calcium, while carbonated beverages can leach calcium from the bones. Maintaining a healthy weight is also important, as being underweight can lead to bone loss, while being overweight can increase the risk of fractures due to falls.

The "Osteoporosis Diet Cookbook for Beginners" aims to simplify the process of adopting a bone-healthy diet by providing a variety of delicious, nutrient-rich recipes. The cookbook is designed to help individuals incorporate bone-strengthening foods into their daily meals effortlessly. Each recipe is crafted to balance the necessary nutrients while ensuring that meals are tasty and easy to prepare. The goal is to make healthy eating a sustainable and enjoyable part of life, thereby supporting long-term bone health.

Living with osteoporosis can be challenging, but with the right dietary choices, it is possible to improve bone density and reduce the risk of fractures. The "Osteoporosis Diet Cookbook for Beginners" serves as a valuable resource for anyone looking to manage or prevent osteoporosis through nutrition. By following the guidelines and recipes in the cookbook, individuals can take proactive steps towards stronger bones and better overall health. Understanding the role of diet in bone health is the first step towards making informed choices that can have a significant impact on quality of life.

What is Osteoporosis?

Osteoporosis is a medical condition characterized by weakened bones, making them fragile and more likely to break. It often progresses without any symptoms until a fracture occurs, which can lead to significant pain and mobility issues. This condition commonly affects older adults, particularly women post-menopause, due to the drop in estrogen levels which plays a crucial role in maintaining bone density. Men are also at risk, especially as they age, but their bone loss tends to occur more gradually. The bones most susceptible to osteoporosis include the hip, spine, and wrist, which can lead to serious health complications if fractures occur.

The development of osteoporosis is influenced by several factors, including genetics, lifestyle choices, and underlying medical conditions. A diet lacking in essential nutrients like calcium and vitamin D, crucial for bone health, significantly increases the risk. Additionally, excessive alcohol consumption, smoking, and a sedentary lifestyle contribute to the deterioration of bone density. Hormonal imbalances, such as those caused by thyroid issues or long-term use of corticosteroids, also play a critical role in the onset of osteoporosis. Understanding these risk factors is essential in preventing and managing the disease.

Nutrition plays a pivotal role in both the prevention and management of osteoporosis. A diet rich in calcium and vitamin D is fundamental to maintaining healthy bones. Calcium is a major component of bone tissue, while vitamin D is essential for the absorption of calcium in the body. Other nutrients like magnesium, vitamin K, and protein also support bone health. Incorporating these nutrients into daily meals can significantly improve bone strength and reduce the risk of fractures. Dairy products, leafy green vegetables, nuts, seeds, and fortified foods are excellent sources of these essential nutrients.

For those diagnosed with osteoporosis or at high risk, the "Osteoporosis Diet Cookbook for Beginners" offers a comprehensive guide to creating meals that support bone health. The cookbook emphasizes foods that are rich in bone-strengthening nutrients and provides recipes that are both delicious and easy to prepare. By following the dietary guidelines outlined in the cookbook, individuals can ensure they are getting the necessary nutrients to support their bone health. The recipes are designed to be balanced, providing a mix of proteins, healthy fats, and carbohydrates, all while prioritizing nutrients that benefit bone density.

Incorporating regular exercise alongside a nutrient-rich diet is crucial for managing osteoporosis. Weight-bearing and resistance exercises stimulate bone formation and improve muscle strength, which helps protect bones from fractures. The cookbook not only provides dietary guidance but also includes lifestyle tips to enhance bone health. Combining a nutritious diet with an active lifestyle creates a holistic approach to managing osteoporosis, reducing the risk of fractures, and improving overall well-being.

Bone health is a long-term commitment, requiring consistent attention to diet and lifestyle. The "Osteoporosis Diet Cookbook for Beginners" serves as a valuable resource, offering practical solutions to integrate bone-healthy foods into everyday life. It simplifies the process of meal planning and preparation, making it easier to adhere to a bone-strengthening diet. This proactive approach empowers individuals to take control of their bone health, preventing the progression of osteoporosis and enhancing their quality of life.

In conclusion, understanding osteoporosis and its relationship with diet is essential for managing and preventing the condition. The "Osteoporosis Diet Cookbook for Beginners" provides the necessary tools and knowledge to create a diet that supports bone health. By incorporating the recipes and tips from the cookbook into daily routines, individuals can significantly reduce their risk of fractures and improve their overall bone strength. This comprehensive guide is not just about food; it's about fostering a healthier, stronger future for those affected by osteoporosis.

Importance of Diet in Managing Osteoporosis

The "Osteoporosis Diet Cookbook for Beginners" emphasizes the profound impact that diet has on managing osteoporosis. Osteoporosis is a condition characterized by weakened bones, making them more susceptible to fractures. Proper nutrition plays a crucial role in strengthening bones and preventing further bone loss. This cookbook provides an essential guide to incorporating bone-healthy foods into everyday meals, making it easier for individuals to manage their condition effectively.

One of the key aspects of an osteoporosis-friendly diet is ensuring an adequate intake of calcium, a mineral vital for bone health. The cookbook offers a variety of recipes rich in calcium, from fortified oatmeal to spinach and feta omelets, ensuring that each meal contributes to building stronger bones. Calcium-rich foods help to replenish the body's calcium reserves, which are often depleted in individuals with osteoporosis, thereby enhancing bone density and reducing the risk of fractures.

Vitamin D is another critical nutrient highlighted in the cookbook, essential for calcium absorption in the body. Without sufficient vitamin D, the body cannot absorb the calcium consumed through diet, rendering it ineffective. The cookbook includes recipes that are not only delicious but also high in vitamin D, such as grilled salmon and fortified cereals. These meals are designed to boost vitamin D levels, aiding in the efficient absorption of calcium and promoting overall bone health.

Protein intake is also addressed in the cookbook, as it plays a significant role in maintaining bone structure. Protein helps in the formation of collagen, a protein that provides a framework for bones. The cookbook includes a range of protein-rich recipes like chicken salad with walnuts and quinoa and black bean salad, ensuring that every meal supports bone strength and repair. Adequate protein intake is particularly important for older adults, whose ability to synthesize protein may decline with age.

The cookbook underscores the importance of magnesium and potassium, minerals that work synergistically with calcium to maintain bone health. Magnesium helps convert vitamin D into its active form, which in turn aids calcium absorption. Potassium neutralizes bone-depleting metabolic acids, helping to preserve bone density. Recipes like lentil soup with kale and stuffed bell peppers with quinoa and turkey are packed with these essential minerals, offering a balanced approach to bone health.

Moreover, the cookbook emphasizes the need to reduce the intake of foods that can negatively impact bone health, such as those high in sodium and caffeine. High sodium levels can lead to calcium loss through urine, while excessive caffeine can interfere with calcium absorption. The recipes in the cookbook are carefully crafted to minimize these elements, promoting a diet that supports bone health without sacrificing flavor. This balanced approach helps individuals manage their osteoporosis more effectively by focusing on foods that nourish rather than deplete bone health.

The "Osteoporosis Diet Cookbook for Beginners" also recognizes the importance of overall dietary patterns in managing osteoporosis. It encourages a varied diet that includes a wide range of fruits, vegetables, whole grains, and lean proteins. This comprehensive approach ensures that individuals receive all the necessary nutrients to support bone health, while also enjoying diverse and satisfying meals. By integrating these dietary principles into daily life, the cookbook offers a sustainable way to improve bone health and overall well-being, making it an invaluable resource for anyone looking to manage osteoporosis through diet.

Chapter 1: Breakfast Recipes

Calcium-Rich Smoothie

Ingredients:

- 1 cup fortified almond milk
- 1/2 cup Greek yogurt
- 1/2 cup frozen spinach
- 1/2 banana
- 1/2 cup frozen berries (blueberries, strawberries, or raspberries)
- 1 tablespoon chia seeds
- 1 teaspoon honey (optional)

Instructions:

1. Combine all ingredients in a blender.
2. Blend on high speed until smooth and creamy.
3. Pour into a glass and serve immediately.

Nutritional Information:

- Calories: 220
- Protein: 10g
- Fat: 5g
- Carbohydrates: 35g
- Fiber: 8g
- Calcium: 450mg

- Vitamin D: 150 IU

Serving Size: 1 smoothie
Cooking Time: 5 minutes

This smoothie is a perfect example of how easy it can be to incorporate bone-healthy foods into your breakfast. The

Spinach and Feta Omelet

Ingredients:

- 2 large eggs
- 1/4 cup of crumbled feta cheese
- 1 cup of fresh spinach, chopped
- 1/4 cup of diced onions
- 1 clove garlic, minced
- 1 tablespoon of olive oil
- Salt and pepper to taste

Instructions:

1. In a bowl, whisk the eggs with a pinch of salt and pepper until well combined.
2. Heat the olive oil in a non-stick skillet over medium heat.
3. Add the onions and garlic, sautéing until they are fragrant and translucent.
4. Add the chopped spinach to the skillet, cooking until it is wilted.
5. Pour the beaten eggs over the spinach and onion mixture, tilting the skillet to spread the eggs evenly.
6. Sprinkle the crumbled feta cheese over the top.
7. Cook the omelet for about 2-3 minutes, until the edges start to set.

8. Carefully fold the omelet in half and cook for another 1-2 minutes, until fully set and the cheese is melted.
9. Serve hot and enjoy!

Nutritional Information:

- Calories: 220
- Protein: 15g
- Fat: 16g
- Carbohydrates: 4g
- Calcium: 200mg
- Vitamin D: 1.5mcg

Serving Size:

- 1 omelet

Cooking Time:

- 10 minutes

Greek Yogurt with Almonds and Berries

Ingredients

- 1 cup plain Greek yogurt
- 1/2 cup fresh berries (strawberries, blueberries, raspberries, or a mix)
- 1/4 cup sliced almonds
- 1 tablespoon honey (optional)
- 1 teaspoon chia seeds (optional)

Instructions

1. Scoop the Greek yogurt into a bowl.
2. Wash and prepare the berries, then add them to the yogurt.
3. Sprinkle sliced almonds over the top.
4. Drizzle with honey if desired for added sweetness.
5. Add chia seeds if using, for an extra nutritional boost.

Nutritional Information

- Calories: 250
- Protein: 20g
- Fat: 10g
- Carbohydrates: 25g

- Calcium: 200mg
- Vitamin C: 15mg

Serving Size
- Serves 1

Cooking Time
- 5 minutes

Fortified Oatmeal with Flaxseeds

Ingredients:

- 1 cup fortified oatmeal
- 2 cups almond milk (calcium-fortified)
- 1 tablespoon flaxseeds
- 1/2 cup fresh berries (blueberries, strawberries, or raspberries)
- 1 tablespoon honey or maple syrup (optional)
- 1/4 teaspoon cinnamon

Instructions:

1. In a medium saucepan, combine the oatmeal and almond milk.
2. Bring to a boil over medium heat, then reduce the heat to low.
3. Simmer for 5-7 minutes, stirring occasionally, until the oatmeal is creamy.
4. Stir in the flaxseeds and cinnamon.
5. Remove from heat and let sit for 1-2 minutes.
6. Serve topped with fresh berries and a drizzle of honey or maple syrup, if desired.

Nutritional Information:

- Calories: 250
- Protein: 8g
- Fat: 6g

- Carbohydrates: 40g
- Fiber: 8g
- Calcium: 300mg
- Vitamin D: 2mcg

Serving Size: 1 bowl

Cooking Time: 10 minutes

Cottage Cheese and Pineapple Bowl

Ingredients:
- 1 cup low-fat cottage cheese
- 1/2 cup fresh pineapple chunks
- 1 tablespoon chia seeds
- 1 tablespoon honey (optional)
- 1/4 teaspoon ground cinnamon

Instructions:
1. Place the cottage cheese in a serving bowl.
2. Add the pineapple chunks on top of the cottage cheese.
3. Sprinkle chia seeds evenly over the bowl.
4. Drizzle honey over the mixture, if using.
5. Sprinkle with ground cinnamon.
6. Mix gently to combine all ingredients.
7. Serve immediately and enjoy.

Nutritional Information:
- Calories: 220
- Protein: 18g
- Carbohydrates: 20g
- Fat: 6g
- Calcium: 250mg

- Vitamin D: 0 IU (consider pairing with a vitamin D supplement or fortified juice)
- Fiber: 4g

Serving Size: 1 bowl
Cooking Time: 5 minutes

Whole Grain Toast with Avocado and Sesame Seeds

Ingredients:

- 2 slices whole grain bread
- 1 ripe avocado
- 1 tablespoon sesame seeds
- Salt and pepper to taste

Instructions:

1. Toast the slices of whole grain bread until golden brown.
2. While the bread is toasting, mash the ripe avocado in a bowl with a fork until smooth.
3. Spread the mashed avocado evenly on top of each slice of toasted bread.
4. Sprinkle sesame seeds over the avocado toast.
5. Season with salt and pepper to taste.
6. Serve immediately.

Nutritional Information:

- Calories: 250
- Protein: 7g
- Carbohydrates: 30g

- Fiber: 10g
- Fat: 12g
- Saturated Fat: 2g
- Sodium: 300mg
- Calcium: 50mg
- Vitamin D: 0IU

Serving Size: 1 serving

Cooking Time: 10 minutes

Chia Seed Pudding with Blueberries

Ingredients:

- 1/4 cup chia seeds
- 1 cup almond milk (or any preferred milk)
- 1 tablespoon honey (optional)
- 1/2 teaspoon vanilla extract
- 1/2 cup fresh blueberries

Instructions:

1. In a bowl, combine chia seeds, almond milk, honey (if using), and vanilla extract. Stir well to mix.
2. Cover the bowl and refrigerate overnight, or for at least 4 hours, to allow the chia seeds to absorb the liquid and thicken.
3. Before serving, stir the pudding to ensure the chia seeds are evenly distributed and have a pudding-like consistency.
4. Top with fresh blueberries before serving.

Nutritional Information:

- Calories: 250
- Total Fat: 12g
  - Saturated Fat: 1g
  - Trans Fat: 0g
- Cholesterol: 0mg
- Sodium: 80mg
- Total Carbohydrates: 29g

- Dietary Fiber: 10g
- Sugars: 12g
- Protein: 7g

Serving Size: 1 serving
Cooking Time: 5 minutes preparation + refrigeration time

Scrambled Eggs with Kale and Mushrooms

Ingredients:

- 2 eggs
- 1 cup chopped kale
- 1/2 cup sliced mushrooms
- Salt and pepper to taste
- 1 teaspoon olive oil

Instructions:

1. Heat olive oil in a non-stick skillet over medium heat.
2. Add mushrooms and sauté until they start to brown.
3. Add chopped kale and cook until wilted.
4. In a bowl, beat eggs with salt and pepper.
5. Pour eggs into the skillet with kale and mushrooms.
6. Stir gently until eggs are cooked through.

Nutritional Information:

- Calories: 250
- Protein: 15g
- Carbohydrates: 6g
- Fat: 18g

- Fiber: 2g
- Calcium: 120mg
- Vitamin D: 6 IU

Serving Size: 1 serving
Cooking Time: 15 minutes

Buckwheat Pancakes with Fresh Fruit

Ingredients:

- 1 cup buckwheat flour
- 1 tablespoon baking powder
- 1/2 teaspoon salt
- 1 tablespoon honey or maple syrup
- 1 cup almond milk (or any milk of choice)
- 1 large egg
- 1 tablespoon melted butter or coconut oil
- Fresh fruit (such as berries, bananas, or peaches) for topping

Instructions:

1. In a large bowl, whisk together buckwheat flour, baking powder, and salt.
2. In another bowl, whisk together honey (or maple syrup), almond milk, egg, and melted butter (or coconut oil).
3. Pour the wet ingredients into the dry ingredients and stir until just combined. Let the batter rest for about 5 minutes.
4. Heat a non-stick skillet or griddle over medium heat. Lightly grease with butter or oil.
5. Pour about 1/4 cup of batter onto the skillet for each pancake. Cook until bubbles form on the surface and the edges look set, about 2-3 minutes. Flip and cook for another 1-2 minutes, or until golden brown.

6. Repeat with the remaining batter. Serve the pancakes topped with fresh fruit.

Nutritional Information:

- Calories: 180
- Total Fat: 6g
- Saturated Fat: 2g
- Cholesterol: 45mg
- Sodium: 360mg
- Total Carbohydrates: 28g
- Dietary Fiber: 3g
- Sugars: 5g
- Protein: 6g

Serving Size: Makes about 8 small pancakes
Cooking Time: About 15 minutes

Quinoa Breakfast Bowl with Nuts and Dried Fruits

Ingredients:

- 1/2 cup quinoa, rinsed
- 1 cup water
- 1/4 cup mixed nuts (almonds, walnuts, pecans)
- 1/4 cup dried fruits (raisins, cranberries, apricots)
- 1 tablespoon honey
- 1/2 teaspoon cinnamon
- Pinch of salt

Instructions:

1. In a small saucepan, bring water to a boil.
2. Add rinsed quinoa and reduce heat to low. Cover and simmer for 15 minutes or until quinoa is tender and water is absorbed.
3. Fluff quinoa with a fork and transfer to a serving bowl.
4. In a separate small pan, toast mixed nuts over medium heat until lightly browned and fragrant, about 3-5 minutes.
5. Add dried fruits, honey, cinnamon, and a pinch of salt to the quinoa. Stir to combine.
6. Top with toasted nuts and dried fruits.
7. Serve warm.

Nutritional Information:

- Calories: 350 kcal
- Protein: 10g
- Carbohydrates: 55g
- Fat: 12g
- Fiber: 7g
- Calcium: 80mg (8% DV)
- Iron: 3mg (17% DV)
- Vitamin D: 0 IU (0% DV)

Serving Size: 1 bowl
Cooking Time: 20 minutes

Chapter 2: Lunch Recipes

Grilled Chicken Salad with Spinach and Walnuts

Ingredients:

- 2 boneless, skinless chicken breasts
- 4 cups fresh spinach leaves
- 1/2 cup walnuts, chopped
- 1/2 cup cherry tomatoes, halved
- 1/4 cup red onion, thinly sliced
- 1/4 cup feta cheese, crumbled
- Salt and pepper to taste
- Olive oil for grilling

Instructions:

1. Preheat grill or grill pan over medium-high heat.
2. Season chicken breasts with salt and pepper, drizzle with olive oil.
3. Grill chicken for 6-7 minutes per side or until cooked through.
4. Remove chicken from grill and let it rest for 5 minutes before slicing.
5. In a large bowl, toss spinach, walnuts, cherry tomatoes, and red onion.

6. Divide salad mixture onto plates, top with sliced chicken and crumbled feta cheese.

Nutritional Information:
- Calories: 350
- Protein: 30g
- Carbohydrates: 9g
- Fat: 22g
- Fiber: 4g
- Calcium: 120mg
- Vitamin D: 5.2mcg

Serving Size: 1 serving
Cooking Time: 15 minutes

Quinoa and Black Bean Salad

Ingredients:

- 1 cup quinoa
- 1 can (15 oz) black beans, rinsed and drained
- 1 red bell pepper, diced
- 1 cup cherry tomatoes, halved
- 1/2 cup red onion, finely chopped
- 1/4 cup fresh cilantro, chopped
- Juice of 1 lime
- 2 tablespoons olive oil
- 1 teaspoon cumin
- Salt and pepper to taste

Instructions:

1. Rinse the quinoa thoroughly under cold water.
2. In a medium saucepan, bring 2 cups of water to a boil.
3. Add the quinoa to the boiling water, cover, and reduce heat to low. Simmer for about 15 minutes or until the quinoa is cooked and the water is absorbed.
4. Fluff the quinoa with a fork and let it cool.
5. In a large bowl, combine the cooked quinoa, black beans, red bell pepper, cherry tomatoes, red onion, and cilantro.

6. In a small bowl, whisk together lime juice, olive oil, cumin, salt, and pepper.

7. Pour the dressing over the salad and toss gently to combine.

8. Serve chilled or at room temperature.

Nutritional Information:

- Calories: 320
- Total Fat: 10g
  - Saturated Fat: 1.5g
  - Trans Fat: 0g
- Cholesterol: 0mg
- Sodium: 280mg
- Total Carbohydrates: 48g
  - Dietary Fiber: 10g
  - Sugars: 3g
- Protein: 12g

Serving Size: Makes 4 servings
Cooking Time: 20 minutes

Salmon and Avocado Wrap

Ingredients:

- 4 oz. grilled salmon fillet
- 1 whole wheat or spinach tortilla wrap
- 1/2 avocado, sliced
- 1/4 cup baby spinach leaves
- 1/4 cup sliced cucumber
- 1 tbsp Greek yogurt
- 1 tsp lemon juice
- Salt and pepper to taste

Instructions:

1. In a small bowl, mix Greek yogurt, lemon juice, salt, and pepper.
2. Lay the tortilla wrap flat and spread the Greek yogurt mixture evenly over it.
3. Layer spinach leaves, cucumber slices, avocado slices, and grilled salmon on top.
4. Roll the tortilla tightly, folding in the sides as you go.
5. Slice the wrap in half diagonally and serve.

- Nutritional Information:

- Calories: 350
- Protein: 25g
- Carbohydrates: 25g

- Fat: 17g
- Fiber: 7g
- Calcium: 100mg
- Vitamin D: 250 IU

Serving Size: 1 wrap

Cooking Time: 15 minutes

Lentil Soup with Kale

Ingredients:

- 1 cup dried lentils, rinsed
- 4 cups vegetable broth
- 1 onion, chopped
- 2 carrots, chopped
- 2 celery stalks, chopped
- 2 garlic cloves, minced
- 1 bay leaf
- 1 tsp dried thyme
- Salt and pepper to taste
- 2 cups chopped kale

Instructions:

1. In a large pot, combine lentils, vegetable broth, onion, carrots, celery, garlic, bay leaf, thyme, salt, and pepper.
2. Bring to a boil, then reduce heat and simmer, covered, for 30-40 minutes or until lentils and vegetables are tender.
3. Stir in chopped kale and cook for an additional 5 minutes until kale is wilted.
4. Remove bay leaf before serving.

Nutritional Information:

- Calories: 250 kcal
- Protein: 15g
- Carbohydrates: 45g
- Fiber: 15g
- Fat: 1g
- Calcium: 80mg (8% DV)
- Vitamin D: 0 IU
- Iron: 4mg (22% DV)

Serving Size: 1 cup
Cooking Time: 45-50 minutes

Chickpea and Tomato Salad

Ingredients:

- 1 can (15 oz) chickpeas, drained and rinsed
- 1 cup cherry tomatoes, halved
- 1/2 cucumber, diced
- 1/4 cup red onion, finely chopped
- 1/4 cup fresh parsley, chopped
- 2 tbsp extra virgin olive oil
- 1 tbsp red wine vinegar
- Salt and pepper to taste

Instructions:

1. In a large bowl, combine chickpeas, cherry tomatoes, cucumber, red onion, and parsley.
2. In a small bowl, whisk together olive oil, red wine vinegar, salt, and pepper.
3. Pour dressing over the salad and toss gently to coat evenly.
4. Refrigerate for at least 30 minutes before serving to allow flavors to meld.

Nutritional Information:

- Serving Size: 1 cup
- Calories: 220
- Total Fat: 10g
  - Saturated Fat: 1g

- Trans Fat: 0g
 - Cholesterol: 0mg
 - Sodium: 290mg
 - Total Carbohydrates: 28g
   - Dietary Fiber: 7g
   - Sugars: 5g
 - Protein: 8g

Cooking Time: 10 minutes

Tofu Stir-Fry with Broccoli and Sesame

Ingredients:

- 1 block firm tofu, drained and cubed
- 2 cups broccoli florets
- 1 red bell pepper, sliced
- 1 tablespoon sesame oil
- 2 tablespoons low-sodium soy sauce
- 1 tablespoon rice vinegar
- 1 tablespoon honey
- 2 cloves garlic, minced
- 1 tablespoon fresh ginger, grated
- Sesame seeds for garnish
- Cooked brown rice or quinoa (optional, for serving)

Instructions:

1. Heat sesame oil in a large skillet over medium heat.
2. Add tofu cubes and cook until golden brown on all sides, about 5-7 minutes. Remove tofu from skillet and set aside.
3. In the same skillet, add broccoli florets and red bell pepper. Stir-fry for 3-4 minutes until vegetables are tender-crisp.
4. In a small bowl, whisk together soy sauce, rice vinegar, honey, garlic, and ginger.
5. Return tofu to the skillet and pour the sauce over the tofu and vegetables. Stir well to coat everything evenly.
6. Cook for another 2-3 minutes until the sauce thickens slightly.

7. Remove from heat and sprinkle with sesame seeds.
8. Serve hot over cooked brown rice or quinoa if desired.

Nutritional Information:

- Calories: 250 per serving
- Protein: 15g
- Fat: 12g
- Carbohydrates: 22g
- Fiber: 5g
- Sodium: 480mg

Serving Size: 1 plate
Cooking Time: 20 minutes

Tuna Salad with Mixed Greens

Ingredients:

- 1 can (5 oz) tuna, drained
- 2 cups mixed greens (spinach, kale, arugula)
- 1/2 cup cherry tomatoes, halved
- 1/4 cucumber, sliced
- 1/4 red onion, thinly sliced
- 1/4 cup sliced almonds
- 1 tablespoon olive oil
- 1 tablespoon balsamic vinegar
- Salt and pepper to taste

Instructions:

1. In a large bowl, combine the mixed greens, cherry tomatoes, cucumber, red onion, and sliced almonds.
2. Add the drained tuna to the salad mixture.
3. Drizzle olive oil and balsamic vinegar over the salad.
4. Season with salt and pepper to taste.
5. Toss gently to combine all ingredients evenly.

Nutritional Information:

- Calories: 320
- Total Fat: 18g

- Saturated Fat: 2g
- Trans Fat: 0g
- Cholesterol: 35mg
- Sodium: 450mg
- Total Carbohydrates: 12g
  - Dietary Fiber: 4g
  - Sugars: 4g
- Protein: 28g

Serving Size: 1 serving
Cooking Time: 15 minutes

Sweet Potato and Black Bean Burrito Bowl

Ingredients:

- 1 sweet potato, peeled and diced
- 1 cup cooked black beans
- 1 cup cooked brown rice
- 1 red bell pepper, diced
- 1/2 cup corn kernels
- 1 avocado, sliced
- 1/4 cup chopped cilantro
- Juice of 1 lime
- Salt and pepper to taste

Instructions:

1. Preheat oven to 400°F (200°C).
2. Toss sweet potato cubes with olive oil, salt, and pepper. Spread on a baking sheet and roast for 20-25 minutes, until tender and lightly browned.
3. In a bowl, combine cooked black beans, brown rice, diced red bell pepper, and corn kernels.
4. To assemble the burrito bowls, divide the rice and bean mixture among serving bowls. Top with roasted sweet potatoes, avocado slices, and chopped cilantro.
5. Drizzle lime juice over each bowl and season with additional salt and pepper to taste.

6. Serve immediately and enjoy!

Nutritional Information:
- Calories: 350
- Protein: 10g
- Carbohydrates: 55g
- Fiber: 12g
- Fat: 12g
- Saturated Fat: 2g
- Sodium: 450mg

Serving Size: 1 bowl
Cooking Time: 30 minutes

Turkey and Swiss Lettuce Wraps

Ingredients:

- 1 lb ground turkey
- 1 tablespoon olive oil
- 1 small onion, diced
- 2 cloves garlic, minced
- 1 teaspoon ground cumin
- 1 teaspoon chili powder
- Salt and pepper to taste
- 1 large tomato, diced
- 1 avocado, sliced
- 4 large lettuce leaves (such as butter lettuce or romaine)
- Optional: salsa or hot sauce for serving

Instructions:

1. Heat olive oil in a large skillet over medium heat. Add diced onion and cook until translucent, about 3-4 minutes.

2. Add minced garlic and cook for another 1-2 minutes until fragrant.

3. Add ground turkey to the skillet, breaking it up with a spatula. Cook until browned and fully cooked through, about 5-7 minutes.

4. Stir in ground cumin, chili powder, salt, and pepper. Cook for an additional 1-2 minutes to allow flavors to meld.

5. Remove skillet from heat and let the turkey mixture cool slightly.

6. To assemble wraps, place a large lettuce leaf on a plate. Spoon turkey mixture onto the leaf.

7. Top with diced tomato and sliced avocado.

8. Optional: drizzle with salsa or hot sauce for added flavor.

9. Roll up the lettuce leaf to enclose the filling, securing with toothpicks if needed.

10. Serve immediately.

Nutritional Information (per serving):

- Calories: 280
- Total Fat: 17g
  - Saturated Fat: 4g
  - Trans Fat: 0g
- Cholesterol: 80mg
- Sodium: 280mg
- Total Carbohydrates: 10g
  - Dietary Fiber: 5g
  - Sugars: 3g
- Protein: 25g

Serving Size: 1 wrap
Cooking Time: 20 minutes

Mediterranean Farro Salad

Ingredients:

- 1 cup farro
- 1 cucumber, diced
- 1 pint cherry tomatoes, halved
- 1/2 cup Kalamata olives, pitted and sliced
- 1/2 cup crumbled feta cheese
- 1/4 cup red onion, finely chopped
- 1/4 cup fresh parsley, chopped
- 1/4 cup extra virgin olive oil
- 2 tablespoons red wine vinegar
- Salt and pepper to taste

Instructions:

1. Cook farro according to package instructions. Drain and let cool.
2. In a large bowl, combine cooled farro, cucumber, cherry tomatoes, olives, feta cheese, red onion, and parsley.
3. In a small bowl, whisk together olive oil, red wine vinegar, salt, and pepper.
4. Pour dressing over salad and toss gently to combine.
5. Serve immediately or refrigerate for flavors to meld.

Nutritional Information:

- Calories: 320 kcal
- Protein: 8g
- Carbohydrates: 35g
- Fat: 16g
- Fiber: 6g
- Sodium: 380mg

Serving Size: 1.5 cups

Cooking Time: 25 minutes

Chapter 3: Dinner Recipes

Baked Cod with Asparagus

Ingredients:

- 4 cod fillets (about 6 ounces each)
- 1 bunch of asparagus, trimmed
- 2 tablespoons olive oil
- 2 cloves garlic, minced
- 1 lemon, sliced
- Salt and pepper to taste

Instructions:

1. Preheat the oven to 400°F (200°C).
2. Place the cod fillets and asparagus on a baking sheet.
3. Drizzle with olive oil and sprinkle minced garlic over the top.
4. Season with salt and pepper.
5. Place lemon slices on top of each cod fillet.
6. Bake for 15-20 minutes, or until the fish flakes easily with a fork and the asparagus is tender.

Nutritional Information:

- Calories: 300 per serving
- Total Fat: 12g
- Saturated Fat: 2g
- Cholesterol: 90mg
- Sodium: 250mg
- Carbohydrates: 8g
- Fiber: 3g
- Sugars: 3g
- Protein: 40g

Serving Size: 1 cod fillet with asparagus
Cooking Time: 20 minutes

Stuffed Bell Peppers with Quinoa and Turkey

Ingredients:

- 4 large bell peppers (any color)
- 1 cup quinoa, rinsed
- 1 lb ground turkey
- 1 onion, diced
- 2 cloves garlic, minced
- 1 can (15 oz) diced tomatoes, drained
- 1 cup spinach, chopped
- 1 tsp dried oregano
- 1 tsp dried basil
- Salt and pepper, to taste
- 1 cup shredded mozzarella cheese (optional)

Instructions:

1. Preheat oven to 375°F (190°C).
2. Cut the tops off the bell peppers and remove seeds and membranes. Place them upright in a baking dish.
3. Cook quinoa according to package instructions.
4. In a large skillet, cook ground turkey over medium heat until browned. Add onion and garlic, cooking until softened.

5. Stir in diced tomatoes, spinach, oregano, basil, salt, and pepper. Cook until spinach is wilted.

6. Remove from heat and stir in cooked quinoa.

7. Spoon the turkey-quinoa mixture evenly into the bell peppers.

8. If desired, sprinkle shredded mozzarella cheese on top of each pepper.

9. Cover the baking dish with foil and bake for 30-35 minutes, or until peppers are tender.

10. Remove foil and bake for an additional 5 minutes to melt cheese (if using).

11. Serve hot and enjoy!

- Nutritional Information (per serving):

- Calories: 350
- Total Fat: 10g
- Saturated Fat: 3g
- Cholesterol: 70mg
- Sodium: 350mg
- Total Carbohydrates: 38g
- Dietary Fiber: 6g
- Sugars: 8g
- Protein: 28g

- **Serving Size:** 1 stuffed pepper
- **Cooking Time:** 1 hour

Spinach and Ricotta Stuffed Chicken Breast

Ingredients:
- 4 boneless, skinless chicken breasts
- 1 cup ricotta cheese
- 1 cup chopped spinach
- 1/2 cup grated Parmesan cheese
- 2 cloves garlic, minced
- Salt and pepper to taste
- Olive oil for cooking

Instructions:
1. Preheat the oven to 375°F (190°C).
2. In a mixing bowl, combine ricotta cheese, chopped spinach, Parmesan cheese, minced garlic, salt, and pepper.
3. Cut a pocket into each chicken breast, being careful not to cut through completely.
4. Stuff each chicken breast with the ricotta and spinach mixture, dividing evenly.
5. Secure the pockets with toothpicks if necessary.
6. Heat olive oil in an oven-safe skillet over medium-high heat.
7. Sear the chicken breasts until golden brown on both sides, about 3-4 minutes per side.

8. Transfer the skillet to the preheated oven and bake for 20-25 minutes, or until the chicken is cooked through and reaches an internal temperature of 165°F (74°C).

9. Remove from the oven and let rest for 5 minutes before serving.

Nutritional Information:

- Calories: 320 per serving
- Total Fat: 15g
  - Saturated Fat: 7g
  - Trans Fat: 0g
- Cholesterol: 120mg
- Sodium: 450mg
- Total Carbohydrates: 4g
  - Dietary Fiber: 1g
  - Sugars: 1g
- Protein: 42g

Serving Size: 1 stuffed chicken breast
Cooking Time: 40-45 minutes

Grilled Salmon with Avocado Salsa

Ingredients:

- 4 salmon fillets
- 2 ripe avocados, diced
- 1/2 red onion, finely chopped
- 1 tomato, diced
- 1 jalapeno, seeded and minced
- Juice of 1 lime
- 2 tablespoons chopped cilantro
- Salt and pepper to taste

Instructions:

1. Preheat grill to medium-high heat.
2. Season salmon fillets with salt and pepper.
3. Grill salmon for 4-5 minutes per side, or until cooked through.
4. In a bowl, combine diced avocado, red onion, tomato, jalapeno, lime juice, cilantro, salt, and pepper to make the avocado salsa.
5. Serve grilled salmon topped with avocado salsa.

Nutritional Information:

- Calories: 350

- Protein: 30g
- Carbohydrates: 10g
- Fat: 20g
- Fiber: 6g

Serving Size: 1 salmon fillet with avocado salsa
Cooking Time: 20 minutes

Beef and Broccoli Stir-Fry

Ingredients:

- 1 lb lean beef, thinly sliced
- 2 cups broccoli florets
- 1 bell pepper, sliced
- 1 onion, thinly sliced
- 3 cloves garlic, minced
- 1 tbsp ginger, minced
- 1/4 cup low-sodium soy sauce
- 2 tbsp oyster sauce
- 1 tbsp cornstarch
- 1 tbsp sesame oil
- 2 tbsp vegetable oil
- Cooked brown rice or whole grain noodles, for serving

Instructions:

1. In a bowl, mix soy sauce, oyster sauce, cornstarch, and sesame oil. Set aside.
2. Heat vegetable oil in a large skillet or wok over medium-high heat.
3. Add beef and stir-fry until browned, about 3-4 minutes. Remove beef and set aside.

4. In the same skillet, add broccoli, bell pepper, onion, garlic, and ginger. Stir-fry for 4-5 minutes until vegetables are tender-crisp.

5. Return beef to the skillet. Pour in the sauce mixture and stir well to coat everything.

6. Cook for another 2-3 minutes until the sauce thickens and everything is heated through.

7. Serve hot over cooked brown rice or whole grain noodles.

Nutritional Information (per serving):

- Calories: 350
- Total Fat: 14g
  - Saturated Fat: 3g
- Cholesterol: 70mg
- Sodium: 800mg
- Total Carbohydrates: 22g
  - Dietary Fiber: 4g
  - Sugars: 5g
- Protein: 32g

Serving Size: 4 servings

Cooking Time: 20 minutes

Baked Eggplant Parmesan

- Ingredients:

- 1 large eggplant, sliced into 1/2-inch rounds
- 1 cup whole wheat breadcrumbs
- 1/2 cup grated Parmesan cheese
- 2 cups marinara sauce
- 1 cup shredded mozzarella cheese
- 2 tablespoons olive oil
- Salt and pepper to taste
- Fresh basil leaves for garnish

- Instructions:

1. Preheat the oven to 400°F (200°C). Grease a baking sheet with olive oil.
2. Arrange the eggplant slices on the baking sheet. Brush both sides of each slice with olive oil and season with salt and pepper.
3. In a shallow dish, combine the breadcrumbs and grated Parmesan cheese.
4. Dredge each eggplant slice in the breadcrumb mixture, coating both sides evenly.
5. Place the coated eggplant slices back onto the baking sheet and bake for 20-25 minutes, or until golden brown and tender.

6. Remove the baking sheet from the oven and reduce the oven temperature to 350°F (175°C).

7. In a baking dish, spread a thin layer of marinara sauce. Arrange half of the baked eggplant slices on top.

8. Spoon more marinara sauce over the eggplant slices and sprinkle with half of the shredded mozzarella cheese.

9. Repeat with another layer of eggplant, marinara sauce, and mozzarella cheese.

10. Cover the baking dish with foil and bake for 20 minutes. Remove the foil and bake for an additional 10 minutes, or until the cheese is bubbly and golden.

11. Garnish with fresh basil leaves before serving.

- **Nutritional Information (per serving):**

- Calories: 350
- Total Fat: 18g
  - Saturated Fat: 7g
- Cholesterol: 25mg
- Sodium: 700mg
- Total Carbohydrates: 32g
  - Dietary Fiber: 7g
  - Total Sugars: 8g
- Protein: 15g

- **Serving Size:** 1/6 of the recipe

- **Cooking Time:** 1 hour

Lemon Garlic Shrimp with Brown Rice

Ingredients:

- 1 lb shrimp, peeled and deveined
- 2 cups brown rice, cooked
- 3 cloves garlic, minced
- 2 tbsp olive oil
- 1 lemon, juiced and zested
- Salt and pepper to taste
- Fresh parsley, chopped (for garnish)

Instructions:

1. Heat olive oil in a large skillet over medium heat. Add minced garlic and sauté until fragrant.
2. Add shrimp to the skillet and cook until they turn pink and opaque, about 3-4 minutes per side.
3. Stir in lemon juice and zest, ensuring shrimp are coated evenly. Season with salt and pepper to taste.
4. Serve the lemon garlic shrimp over cooked brown rice, garnished with chopped parsley.

Nutritional Information:

- Calories: 320
- Protein: 25g

- Carbohydrates: 35g
- Fat: 10g
- Fiber: 3g
- Calcium: 50mg
- Vitamin D: 2.5mcg

Serving Size: 1 plate

Cooking Time: 20 minutes

Pork Tenderloin with Apple Slaw

Ingredients:

- 1 pork tenderloin (about 1 lb)
- 2 apples, thinly sliced
- 1 cup shredded cabbage
- 1/4 cup shredded carrots
- 2 tablespoons apple cider vinegar
- 1 tablespoon honey
- Salt and pepper to taste

Instructions:

1. Preheat oven to 400°F (200°C).
2. Season pork tenderloin with salt and pepper.
3. Place pork tenderloin on a baking sheet and roast for 25-30 minutes, or until internal temperature reaches 145°F (63°C).
4. In a bowl, combine sliced apples, shredded cabbage, shredded carrots, apple cider vinegar, honey, salt, and pepper. Mix well to coat evenly.
5. Let the pork rest for 5 minutes before slicing. Serve with apple slaw on the side.

Nutritional Information:

- Calories: 300

- Protein: 30g
- Carbohydrates: 20g
- Fat: 10g
- Fiber: 4g
- Calcium: 30mg
- Vitamin D: 2mcg

Serving Size: 4 servings

Cooking Time: 30 minutes

Vegetable and Chickpea Curry

- Ingredients:

- 1 tablespoon olive oil
- 1 onion, finely chopped
- 2 garlic cloves, minced
- 1 tablespoon ginger, grated
- 1 teaspoon ground turmeric
- 1 teaspoon ground cumin
- 1 teaspoon ground coriander
- 1/2 teaspoon chili powder (adjust to taste)
- 1 can (15 ounces) chickpeas, drained and rinsed
- 1 can (14 ounces) diced tomatoes
- 1 can (14 ounces) coconut milk
- 2 cups cauliflower florets
- 1 cup spinach leaves
- Salt and pepper to taste
- Fresh cilantro, chopped (for garnish)

- Instructions:

1. Heat olive oil in a large skillet over medium heat. Add chopped onion and sauté until translucent, about 5 minutes.
2. Add minced garlic and grated ginger, cook for another 1-2 minutes until fragrant.

3. Stir in ground turmeric, cumin, coriander, and chili powder. Cook for 1 minute to toast the spices.

4. Add chickpeas, diced tomatoes (with juices), and coconut milk to the skillet. Stir well to combine.

5. Bring the mixture to a simmer, then add cauliflower florets. Cover and cook for 10-15 minutes, or until cauliflower is tender.

6. Stir in spinach leaves and cook for an additional 2-3 minutes until wilted.

7. Season with salt and pepper to taste. Garnish with chopped cilantro before serving.

- **Nutritional Information:**

- Calories: 320 kcal
- Protein: 10g
- Carbohydrates: 30g
- Fat: 20g
- Fiber: 8g
- Sodium: 480mg

- **Serving Size:** 4 servings

- **Cooking Time:** 30 minutes

Mushroom and Barley Risotto

Ingredients:

- 1 cup pearl barley
- 4 cups low-sodium vegetable broth
- 1 tablespoon olive oil
- 1 onion, finely chopped
- 2 cloves garlic, minced
- 8 oz cremini mushrooms, sliced
- 1/2 cup dry white wine
- 1/2 cup grated Parmesan cheese
- Salt and pepper to taste
- Fresh parsley, chopped (for garnish)

Instructions:

1. In a saucepan, bring the vegetable broth to a simmer and keep it warm.
2. In a separate large skillet, heat olive oil over medium heat. Add onion and garlic, sauté until softened.
3. Add mushrooms and cook until they release their juices and start to brown.
4. Stir in pearl barley and cook for 1-2 minutes until toasted.
5. Pour in the white wine and cook until it is absorbed, stirring frequently.

6. Begin adding the warm vegetable broth, one ladleful at a time, stirring frequently and allowing each addition to be absorbed before adding the next.
7. Continue cooking until the barley is tender and creamy, about 30-40 minutes.
8. Stir in grated Parmesan cheese and season with salt and pepper to taste.
9. Remove from heat and let it sit for a few minutes to thicken.
10. Serve hot, garnished with fresh chopped parsley.

Nutritional Information:

- Calories: 320 kcal
- Protein: 12g
- Carbohydrates: 52g
- Fat: 7g
- Sodium: 480mg
- Fiber: 10g

Serving Size: 1 cup
Cooking Time: 45 minutes

Chapter 4: Desserts

Baked Apples with Cinnamon

- Ingredients:
- 4 medium apples (such as Granny Smith or Honeycrisp)
- 2 tablespoons honey or maple syrup
- 1 teaspoon ground cinnamon
- 1/4 cup chopped walnuts or almonds (optional)

- Instructions:
1. Preheat the oven to 375°F (190°C).
2. Core the apples, leaving the bottom intact. Place them in a baking dish.
3. Drizzle honey or maple syrup over the apples, then sprinkle with cinnamon.
4. If desired, stuff each apple with chopped nuts.
5. Bake for 25-30 minutes, or until the apples are tender.
6. Serve warm, optionally topped with a dollop of Greek yogurt or a sprinkle of additional cinnamon.

Nutritional Information (per serving):

- Calories: 150
- Total Fat: 3g
- Saturated Fat: 0g
- Cholesterol: 0mg
- Sodium: 0mg
- Total Carbohydrates: 32g
- Dietary Fiber: 5g
- Sugars: 24g
- Protein: 1g

Serving Size: 1 baked apple
Cooking Time: 25-30 minutes

Chia Seed Pudding with Mango

- Ingredients:

- 1/4 cup chia seeds
- 1 cup unsweetened almond milk (or milk of choice)
- 1 tablespoon honey or maple syrup (optional, to taste)
- 1 ripe mango, diced
- Fresh berries (optional, for garnish)

- Instructions:

1. In a bowl, combine chia seeds and almond milk. Stir well to mix.
2. Add honey or maple syrup if desired for sweetness.
3. Let the mixture sit for 10 minutes, then stir again to break up any clumps of chia seeds.
4. Cover and refrigerate for at least 2 hours or overnight, allowing the chia seeds to absorb the liquid and thicken.
5. Before serving, stir the pudding to ensure a smooth consistency.
6. Divide the pudding into serving bowls or glasses.
7. Top each serving with diced mango and fresh berries, if using, for added flavor and nutrition.

- Nutritional Information (per serving):

- Calories: 180 kcal
- Protein: 4g
- Carbohydrates: 26g
- Fiber: 10g
- Sugars: 14g
- Fat: 7g
- Saturated Fat: 1g
- Cholesterol: 0mg
- Sodium: 100mg
- Calcium: 300mg
- Vitamin D: 120 IU

- **Serving Size**: 1 serving
- **Cooking Time:** 10 minutes preparation + 2 hours refrigeration

Dark Chocolate Almond Bark

Ingredients:
- 8 oz dark chocolate (at least 70% cocoa)
- 1/2 cup almonds, chopped
- Sea salt, to taste

Instructions:
1. Line a baking sheet with parchment paper.
2. Melt the dark chocolate in a microwave-safe bowl in 30-second intervals, stirring in between until smooth.
3. Spread the melted chocolate evenly onto the prepared baking sheet.
4. Sprinkle chopped almonds over the melted chocolate, pressing them gently into the surface.
5. Sprinkle with sea salt for added flavor.
6. Place the baking sheet in the refrigerator for about 30 minutes, or until the chocolate hardens.
7. Once hardened, break the bark into pieces.
8. Store in an airtight container in the refrigerator.

Nutritional Information:
- Serving Size: 1 ounce
- Calories: 150

- Total Fat: 10g
  - Saturated Fat: 4g
  - Trans Fat: 0g
- Cholesterol: 0mg
- Sodium: 5mg
- Total Carbohydrate: 15g
  - Dietary Fiber: 3g
  - Sugars: 9g
- Protein: 3g

- **Cooking Time:** 10 minutes

Berry Yogurt Popsicles

Ingredients:
- 1 cup mixed berries (such as strawberries, blueberries, raspberries)
- 1 cup plain Greek yogurt
- 1 tablespoon honey (optional)
- Popsicle molds and sticks

Instructions:
1. Wash and chop the berries as needed.
2. In a blender or food processor, combine the berries, Greek yogurt, and honey (if using). Blend until smooth.
3. Pour the mixture into popsicle molds, leaving a little space at the top for expansion.
4. Insert popsicle sticks into each mold.
5. Freeze for at least 4 hours or until completely firm.
6. To remove the popsicles from the molds, briefly run warm water over the outside of the molds.
7. Serve immediately and enjoy!

Nutritional Information:
- Calories: 60 per serving
- Protein: 5g

- Carbohydrates: 10g
- Fat: 0.5g
- Fiber: 2g
- Calcium: 100mg (10% DV)
- Vitamin C: 15mg (25% DV)

Serving Size: Makes 6 popsicles
Cooking Time: 10 minutes preparation + 4 hours freezing

Oatmeal Raisin Cookies

Ingredients:

- 1 cup old-fashioned oats
- 1/2 cup whole wheat flour
- 1/2 teaspoon baking soda
- 1/2 teaspoon ground cinnamon
- 1/4 teaspoon salt
- 1/4 cup unsalted butter, softened
- 1/4 cup honey or maple syrup
- 1 large egg
- 1 teaspoon vanilla extract
- 1/2 cup raisins

Instructions:

1. Preheat oven to 350°F (175°C). Line a baking sheet with parchment paper.
2. In a bowl, whisk together oats, flour, baking soda, cinnamon, and salt.
3. In another bowl, cream together butter and honey/maple syrup until smooth. Beat in egg and vanilla extract.
4. Gradually add dry ingredients to wet ingredients, mixing until well combined. Fold in raisins.

5. Drop tablespoonfuls of dough onto the prepared baking sheet, spacing them about 2 inches apart. Flatten each cookie slightly with a fork.

6. Bake for 10-12 minutes, or until edges are golden brown.

7. Allow cookies to cool on the baking sheet for 5 minutes before transferring to a wire rack to cool completely.

Nutritional Information:

- Serving Size: 1 cookie
- Calories: 120
- Total Fat: 5g
  - Saturated Fat: 2.5g
- Cholesterol: 20mg
- Sodium: 80mg
- Total Carbohydrates: 18g
  - Dietary Fiber: 2g
  - Sugars: 7g
- Protein: 2g

Cooking Time: 10-12 minutes

Conclusion

The conclusion of the "Osteoporosis Diet Cookbook for Beginners" encapsulates the journey towards better bone health through informed dietary choices. It serves as a summary of the key principles and benefits outlined throughout the cookbook, reinforcing the importance of a bone-healthy diet in managing osteoporosis.

In this final section, readers are reminded of the fundamental role that nutrition plays in maintaining strong bones and preventing fractures. The cookbook emphasizes the consumption of calcium-rich foods, such as dairy products, leafy greens, and fortified cereals, which are essential for bone strength. It also underscores the significance of vitamin D in aiding calcium absorption, highlighting the inclusion of vitamin D-rich foods like fatty fish and fortified dairy alternatives.

Furthermore, the conclusion of the cookbook reinforces the holistic approach to bone health, which includes not only diet but also exercise and lifestyle adjustments. It encourages readers to engage in weight-bearing exercises, such as walking, jogging, or resistance training, which help to build and maintain bone density. Additionally, the importance of sunlight exposure for natural vitamin D synthesis is emphasized, alongside the recommendation to avoid smoking and excessive alcohol consumption, which can negatively impact bone health.

The conclusion serves as a call to action, urging readers to implement the knowledge gained from the cookbook into their daily lives. It encourages them to create personalized meal plans based on the provided recipes and nutritional guidelines, ensuring that every meal supports their journey towards stronger bones and overall well-being. By adopting these practices, individuals can proactively manage their osteoporosis and reduce the risk of bone-related complications.

Ultimately, the conclusion of the "Osteoporosis Diet Cookbook for Beginners" instills confidence and empowerment in its readers. It reassures them that with dedication to a balanced and nutritious diet, supported by the practical insights and recipes within the cookbook, they can effectively enhance their bone health and enjoy a fulfilling lifestyle. This final section serves as a fitting conclusion to a comprehensive guide that not only educates but also empowers individuals to take charge of their health and well-being through informed dietary choices.

www.ingramcontent.com/pod-product-compliance
Lightning Source LLC
Chambersburg PA
CBHW072052230526
45479CB00010B/848